CONGENITAL CONDITIONS AND INBORN ERRORS OF METABOLISM

150 Clinical Questions

Dr Essam Abdelhakim

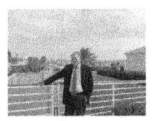

Copyright © 2024 Dr Essam Abdelhakim

All rights reserved

The characters and events portrayed in this book are fictitious. Any similarity to real persons, living or dead, is coincidental and not intended by the author.

No part of this book may be reproduced, or stored in a retrieval system, or transmitted in any form or by any means, electronic, mechanical, photocopying, recording, or otherwise, without express written permission of the publisher.

Cover design by: Art Painter
Library of Congress Control Number: 2018675309
Printed in the United States of America

CONTENTS

Title Page
Copyright
Disclosure
Introduction   1
Questions&Answers   3
About The Author   65

DISCLOSURE

Disclosure

This book has been created with the assistance of *Artificial Intelligence (AI) tools* and thoroughly reviewed and edited by the author to ensure clarity, relevance, and educational value.

While every effort has been made to provide accurate and up-to-date information, this content is intended solely for educational and informational purposes.

The author is a medical professional; however, the information provided in this book *is not a substitute for professional medical advice, diagnosis, or treatment.*

Readers are strongly advised to consult licensed healthcare providers or specialists for any medical concerns or conditions.

By using this book, **you acknowledge and agree** that the author shall not be held responsible or liable for any loss, damage, or harm whether physical, emotional, financial, or otherwise that may occur *as a result of the use or misuse of the information presented herein.*

INTRODUCTION

Congenital anomalies and inborn errors of metabolism represent a significant area of concern in pediatric medicine, with profound implications for diagnosis, management, and long-term outcomes. These conditions are diverse, ranging from structural malformations evident at birth to subtle metabolic defects that may manifest later in life. Understanding these disorders is critical for medical students, residents, and healthcare providers tasked with recognizing, diagnosing, and treating affected individuals.

This book is designed to serve as a comprehensive resource for mastering key concepts related to congenital anomalies and inborn errors of metabolism. By combining high-yield multiple-choice questions with detailed explanations, we aim to enhance understanding and retention of this essential material. The topics covered include:

- Fundamental principles of embryology and pathophysiology of congenital anomalies
- Diagnostic techniques and approaches
- Common and rare inborn errors of metabolism
- Key aspects of management and treatment options

Each chapter provides insights into the underlying mechanisms, clinical presentations, and evidence-based interventions for these conditions. Additionally, pearls of wisdom are included to highlight critical take-home points and facilitate application in clinical practice. Designed to support medical students preparing for exams as well as clinicians seeking to refine their knowledge, this book ensures a thorough grounding in this complex and rapidly evolving field.

Let us embark on this journey to explore the fascinating intricacies of congenital anomalies and inborn errors of metabolism, equipping ourselves to deliver the best possible care for our patients.

QUESTIONS&ANSWERS

1. **Which congenital anomaly is associated with maternal folate deficiency?**
    - A) Cleft palate
    - B) Neural tube defects
    - C) Congenital diaphragmatic hernia
    - D) Tetralogy of Fallot

    Answer: B
    Explanation: Neural tube defects such as spina bifida and anencephaly are linked to folate deficiency. Folic acid supplementation during pregnancy reduces the risk.

2. **What is the most sensitive screening test for neural tube defects during pregnancy?**
    - A) Chorionic villus sampling
    - B) Amniotic fluid acetylcholinesterase levels
    - C) Maternal serum alpha-fetoprotein (MSAFP)
    - D) Fetal ultrasound

    Answer: C
    Explanation: Elevated maternal serum alpha-fetoprotein (MSAFP) is the most sensitive screening test for neural tube defects.

3. **Which type of spina bifida is characterized by a visible cystic mass containing meninges and cerebrospinal fluid?**
    - A) Spina bifida occulta

- B) Meningocele
- C) Myelomeningocele
- D) Rachischisis

Answer: B

Explanation: Meningocele presents as a cystic mass containing meninges and cerebrospinal fluid, but no neural tissue. Myelomeningocele includes neural tissue.

4. **Which of the following is a common complication of myelomeningocele?**
   - A) Hydrocephalus
   - B) Duodenal atresia
   - C) Microcephaly
   - D) Esophageal atresia

   Answer: A

   Explanation: Hydrocephalus often develops due to Arnold-Chiari malformation associated with myelomeningocele.

5. **What is the primary prevention strategy for neural tube defects?**
   - A) Vitamin D supplementation
   - B) Maternal immunization
   - C) Folic acid supplementation
   - D) Regular exercise

   Answer: C

   Explanation: Daily folic acid supplementation of 400-800 µg before and during pregnancy significantly reduces the risk of neural tube defects.

6. **Which congenital heart defect is most commonly associated with Down syndrome?**
   - A) Tetralogy of Fallot

- B) Ventricular septal defect
- C) Atrioventricular septal defect
- D) Patent ductus arteriosus

Answer: C

Explanation: Atrioventricular septal defects are highly associated with Down syndrome.

7. **A newborn presents with cyanosis that worsens with feeding but improves with crying. What is the most likely diagnosis?**
    - A) Tetralogy of Fallot
    - B) Transposition of the great arteries
    - C) Choanal atresia
    - D) Truncus arteriosus

    Answer: C

    Explanation: Cyanosis that improves with crying is a hallmark of choanal atresia.

8. **What is the initial treatment for a newborn with transposition of the great arteries?**
    - A) Balloon atrial septostomy
    - B) Administration of prostaglandin E1
    - C) Surgical correction
    - D) Beta-blockers

    Answer: B

    Explanation: Prostaglandin E1 maintains ductal patency, which is critical for survival until definitive surgical correction.

9. **What is the characteristic finding on chest X-ray in a patient with tetralogy of Fallot?**
    - A) Boot-shaped heart
    - B) Egg-on-string appearance
    - C) Snowman appearance
    - D) Figure-of-eight sign

Answer: A

Explanation: The boot-shaped heart is due to right ventricular hypertrophy in tetralogy of Fallot.

10. **Which of the following is NOT a component of tetralogy of Fallot?**
    - A) Pulmonary stenosis
    - B) Right ventricular hypertrophy
    - C) Overriding aorta
    - D) Left ventricular hypertrophy

    Answer: D

    Explanation: Tetralogy of Fallot includes pulmonary stenosis, right ventricular hypertrophy, ventricular septal defect, and overriding aorta.

11. **What is the primary difference between omphalocele and gastroschisis?**
    - A) Location of the defect
    - B) Presence of a sac covering the intestines
    - C) Association with chromosomal abnormalities
    - D) Size of the defect

    Answer: B

    Explanation: Omphalocele involves a sac covering the intestines, while gastroschisis does not. Omphalocele is more commonly associated with chromosomal abnormalities.

12. **Which abdominal wall defect is more likely to be associated with other congenital anomalies?**
    - A) Gastroschisis
    - B) Omphalocele

- C) Umbilical hernia
- D) Diastasis recti

Answer: B

Explanation: Omphalocele is frequently associated with other anomalies, such as cardiac or chromosomal defects.

13. **Which imaging modality is most useful in diagnosing abdominal wall defects prenatally?**
    - A) MRI
    - B) Ultrasound
    - C) CT scan
    - D) X-ray

    Answer: B

    Explanation: Prenatal ultrasound is the most effective tool for detecting abdominal wall defects.

14. **What is the recommended management for a neonate with gastroschisis?**
    - A) Immediate surgical repair
    - B) Antibiotics only
    - C) Delayed surgical repair
    - D) Observation

    Answer: A

    Explanation: Gastroschisis requires immediate surgical repair to protect the exposed intestines and prevent infection.

15. **Which of the following is NOT a complication of untreated omphalocele?**
    - A) Hypothermia
    - B) Hypoglycemia
    - C) Respiratory distress
    - D) Hypertension

Answer: D
Explanation: Untreated omphalocele can lead to complications such as hypothermia, hypoglycemia, and respiratory distress, but not hypertension.

16. **Which of the following is the most common amino acid metabolism disorder?**
    - A) Phenylketonuria (PKU)
    - B) Maple syrup urine disease
    - C) Homocystinuria
    - D) Alkaptonuria

    Answer: A
    Explanation: PKU is the most common amino acid disorder, caused by phenylalanine hydroxylase deficiency.

17. **A child presents with developmental delay and a musty body odor. Which test is diagnostic?**
    - A) Serum ammonia levels
    - B) Plasma amino acid analysis
    - C) Urinary organic acid analysis
    - D) Serum lactate levels

    Answer: B
    Explanation: Plasma amino acid analysis reveals elevated phenylalanine in PKU.

18. **What is the dietary restriction for a patient with PKU?**
    - A) Avoidance of branched-chain amino acids
    - B) Avoidance of phenylalanine
    - C) Avoidance of methionine
    - D) Avoidance of tyrosine

    Answer: B

Explanation: Phenylalanine must be restricted in PKU to prevent neurotoxicity.

19. **Which cofactor is often supplemented in patients with atypical PKU?**
    - A) Biotin
    - B) Pyridoxine
    - C) Tetrahydrobiopterin (BH4)
    - D) Thiamine

    Answer: C

    Explanation: BH4 deficiency causes atypical PKU, and supplementation can improve outcomes.

20. **What is the inheritance pattern of PKU?**
    - A) X-linked recessive
    - B) Autosomal dominant
    - C) Autosomal recessive
    - D) Mitochondrial

    Answer: C

    Explanation: PKU is inherited in an autosomal recessive manner.

21. **A neonate develops jaundice, hepatomegaly, and vomiting after consuming breast milk. What is the likely diagnosis?**
    - A) Phenylketonuria
    - B) Galactosemia
    - C) Maple syrup urine disease
    - D) Homocystinuria

    Answer: B

    Explanation: Galactosemia results from deficiency in galactose-1-phosphate uridyltransferase, leading to toxic metabolite accumulation.

22. What are the typical ultrasound findings associated with spina bifida during prenatal screening?

- A. Lemon sign and banana sign
- B. Double bubble sign
- C. Sandal gap deformity
- D. Strawberry-shaped skull

Answer: A. Lemon sign and banana sign

Explanation: On prenatal ultrasound, the lemon sign refers to the scalloping of the frontal bones, and the banana sign refers to the cerebellum's shape due to downward displacement. These are hallmark signs of spina bifida and Chiari II malformation.

Pearl: Early diagnosis allows for better counseling and planning of potential in-utero surgical interventions.

23. What dietary restriction is critical for managing phenylketonuria (PKU)?

- A. Low-sodium diet
- B. Low-phenylalanine diet
- C. High-protein diet
- D. Gluten-free diet

Answer: B. Low-phenylalanine diet

Explanation: Phenylketonuria is caused by a deficiency in phenylalanine hydroxylase, leading to an accumulation of phenylalanine, which can cause severe intellectual disability. A diet low in phenylalanine, avoiding high-protein foods like meat, dairy, and certain grains, is essential.

Pearl: Early detection through newborn screening and dietary management can prevent the neurological sequelae of PKU.

24. Which congenital anomaly is most commonly associated with oligohydramnios?

- A. Potter sequence

- B. Tetralogy of Fallot
- C. Gastroschisis
- D. Congenital diaphragmatic hernia

Answer: A. Potter sequence

Explanation: Oligohydramnios, or reduced amniotic fluid, is often linked to renal agenesis or urinary tract obstruction. The lack of amniotic fluid results in compression of the fetus, leading to characteristic facial anomalies, limb deformities, and pulmonary hypoplasia.

Pearl: Early identification of oligohydramnios warrants evaluation of renal function and fetal anatomy.

25. What is the genetic inheritance pattern of cystic fibrosis (CF)?

- A. X-linked recessive
- B. Autosomal dominant
- C. Autosomal recessive
- D. Mitochondrial inheritance

Answer: C. Autosomal recessive

Explanation: Cystic fibrosis is caused by mutations in the CFTR gene on chromosome 7. Both parents must be carriers of the defective gene for the condition to manifest in their offspring.

Pearl: CF is the most common lethal genetic disorder among Caucasians, with newborn screening programs aiding early diagnosis and treatment.

26. Which metabolic disorder presents with a "mousy" odor?

- A. Maple syrup urine disease
- B. Phenylketonuria
- C. Homocystinuria
- D. Tyrosinemia

Answer: B. Phenylketonuria

Explanation: The "mousy" or musty odor in PKU is due to the accumulation of phenylacetic acid, a metabolite of phenylalanine. This distinctive odor can be a clue to diagnosis.

Pearl: Routine newborn screening for PKU is critical for early identification and management.

27. What congenital cardiac anomaly is most associated with Down syndrome?

- A. Atrioventricular septal defect (AVSD)
- B. Tetralogy of Fallot
- C. Patent ductus arteriosus
- D. Coarctation of the aorta

Answer: A. Atrioventricular septal defect (AVSD)

Explanation: Approximately 40-50% of children with Down syndrome have congenital heart defects, with AVSD being the most common. It results from incomplete fusion of the endocardial cushions.

Pearl: Early echocardiographic evaluation is essential for all newborns with Down syndrome to assess for heart defects.

28. Which of the following is a common feature of Marfan syndrome?

- A. Blue sclera
- B. Lens dislocation (ectopia lentis)
- C. Macroglossia
- D. Cafe-au-lait spots

Answer: B. Lens dislocation (ectopia lentis)

Explanation: Marfan syndrome, caused by mutations in the FBN1 gene, often presents with ectopia lentis, characterized by the upward dislocation of the lens. Other features include aortic root dilation, long extremities, and joint hypermobility.

Pearl: Annual ophthalmologic and cardiovascular evaluations are critical for managing complications in Marfan syndrome.

29. What is the hallmark biochemical finding in Tay-Sachs disease?
- A. Increased homogentisic acid
- B. Elevated ammonia levels
- C. Accumulation of GM2 ganglioside
- D. Decreased alpha-fetoprotein

Answer: C. Accumulation of GM2 ganglioside

Explanation: Tay-Sachs disease is caused by a deficiency of the enzyme hexosaminidase A, leading to the accumulation of GM2 ganglioside in neurons. This results in progressive neurodegeneration, developmental delay, and the classic cherry-red macula.

Pearl: Genetic counseling is important in populations with a higher prevalence of Tay-Sachs, such as Ashkenazi Jews.

30. What is the primary treatment for urea cycle disorders?
- A. High-protein diet
- C. Ketogenic diet
- D. Bone marrow transplantation

Answer: B. Low-protein diet and ammonia-scavenging agents

Explanation: Urea cycle disorders result in the accumulation of ammonia, which is neurotoxic. Management includes reducing protein intake to decrease ammonia production and using medications like sodium phenylbutyrate to facilitate ammonia excretion.

Pearl: Early diagnosis and treatment can prevent catastrophic hyperammonemia, particularly in newborns.

31. Which congenital anomaly results from failure of the foregut to divide into the esophagus and trachea?

- A. Gastroschisis
- B. Diaphragmatic hernia
- C. Tracheoesophageal fistula
- D. Omphalocele

Answer: C. Tracheoesophageal fistula

Explanation: Tracheoesophageal fistula (TEF) often presents shortly after birth with drooling, choking, and respiratory distress when feeding. It results from incomplete separation of the esophagus and trachea during embryogenesis.

Pearl: The "VACTERL" association (Vertebral, Anorectal, Cardiac, Tracheoesophageal, Renal, and Limb anomalies) should be considered when TEF is identified.

32. Which congenital anomaly is characterized by the absence of the cranial vault and most of the brain?

- A. Encephalocele
- B. Anencephaly
- C. Holoprosencephaly
- D. Microcephaly

Answer: B. Anencephaly

Explanation: Anencephaly is a neural tube defect that results in the absence of a major portion of the brain, skull, and scalp. It occurs due to failure of the neural tube to close at the cranial end during early embryogenesis.

Pearl: Adequate folic acid supplementation before and during pregnancy significantly reduces the risk of neural tube defects like anencephaly.

33. What is the hallmark biochemical abnormality in maple syrup urine disease (MSUD)?

- A. Increased phenylalanine levels
- B. Increased glycine levels
- C. Increased branched-chain amino acids (leucine,

isoleucine, valine)
- D. Decreased lysine levels

Answer: C. Increased branched-chain amino acids (leucine, isoleucine, valine)

Explanation: MSUD is caused by a deficiency in branched-chain alpha-keto acid dehydrogenase complex, leading to the accumulation of branched-chain amino acids and their toxic metabolites. The disease is named for the distinctive maple syrup odor of the urine.

Pearl: Early diagnosis through newborn screening and dietary restriction of branched-chain amino acids can prevent severe neurological complications.

34. Which syndrome is associated with congenital absence of the thymus and parathyroid glands?
- A. Turner syndrome
- B. DiGeorge syndrome
- C. Williams syndrome
- D. Klinefelter syndrome

Answer: B. DiGeorge syndrome

Explanation: DiGeorge syndrome (22q11.2 deletion syndrome) results in developmental defects of the third and fourth pharyngeal pouches, leading to hypoplasia or absence of the thymus and parathyroid glands. This results in immunodeficiency and hypocalcemia.

Pearl: Immunological evaluation and calcium monitoring are critical in managing patients with DiGeorge syndrome.

35. Which inborn error of metabolism presents with cataracts in the first few weeks of life?
- A. Galactosemia
- B. Phenylketonuria

- C. Homocystinuria
- D. Tyrosinemia

Answer: A. Galactosemia

Explanation: Galactosemia is caused by a deficiency of galactose-1-phosphate uridyltransferase, leading to the accumulation of galactose and its metabolites. These metabolites can cause cataracts, hepatomegaly, and intellectual disability if untreated.

Pearl: Eliminating lactose and galactose from the diet can prevent complications in galactosemia.

36. What is the characteristic facial feature in fetal alcohol syndrome?

- A. Epicanthal folds
- B. Smooth philtrum
- C. Large ears
- D. Wide nasal bridge

Answer: B. Smooth philtrum

Explanation: Fetal alcohol syndrome is characterized by a smooth philtrum, thin upper lip, and small palpebral fissures. These features, along with growth retardation and neurodevelopmental abnormalities, are due to prenatal alcohol exposure.

Pearl: Early intervention and supportive therapies can help manage developmental delays associated with fetal alcohol syndrome.

37. In the differential diagnosis of an infant with jaundice and hepatic dysfunction, which of the following inborn errors of metabolism should be considered?

a) Galactosemia
b) Hereditary tyrosinemia
c) Neonatal hemochromatosis
d) All of the above

Answer: d) All of the above

Explanation: Jaundice or other evidence of hepatic dysfunction can be the mode of presentation for several inborn errors of metabolism, including galactosemia, hereditary tyrosinemia, and neonatal hemochromatosis

38. Which amino acid accumulates in maple syrup urine disease?
- A. Tyrosine
- B. Leucine
- C. Arginine
- D. Lysine

Answer: B. Leucine

Explanation: Maple syrup urine disease results from a defect in branched-chain alpha-keto acid dehydrogenase, leading to the accumulation of leucine, isoleucine, and valine. The disease is characterized by sweet-smelling urine and severe neurological symptoms if untreated.

Pearl: Early dietary intervention with restriction of branched-chain amino acids is critical for preventing neurologic damage.

39. Which enzyme deficiency causes galactosemia?
- A. Galactose-1-phosphate uridyltransferase (GALT)
- B. Glucose-6-phosphatase
- C. Hexokinase
- D. Fructokinase

Answer: A. Galactose-1-phosphate uridyltransferase (GALT)

Explanation: GALT deficiency impairs galactose metabolism, resulting in toxic accumulation of galactose-1-phosphate. Symptoms include jaundice, hepatomegaly, cataracts, and developmental delay.

Pearl: Newborn screening allows for early identification and dietary management by excluding galactose-containing foods such as milk.

40. Which metabolic disorder presents with a "sweaty feet" odor?
- A. Homocystinuria
- B. Tyrosinemia type I
- **C. Isovaleric acidemia**
- D. Phenylketonuria

Answer: C. Isovaleric acidemia

Explanation: Isovaleric acidemia is caused by a deficiency of isovaleryl-CoA dehydrogenase, leading to the accumulation of isovaleric acid. This disorder presents with metabolic acidosis, lethargy, and the characteristic "sweaty feet" odor.

Pearl: Management includes dietary protein restriction and carnitine supplementation.

41. What is the primary treatment for methylmalonic acidemia?
- A. Hemodialysis
- B. Vitamin B12 supplementation
- C. Corticosteroids
- D. Insulin therapy

Answer: B. Vitamin B12 supplementation

Explanation: Methylmalonic acidemia can result from vitamin B12 deficiency or a defect in the enzyme methylmalonyl-CoA mutase. Patients benefit from B12 supplementation, dietary management, and addressing metabolic crises.

Pearl: Acute decompensation in methylmalonic acidemia can lead to severe acidosis and hyperammonemia, requiring urgent intervention.

CONGENITAL CONDITIONS AND INBORN ERRORS OF METABOLISM

42. Which inborn error of metabolism can lead to early cataract formation?

- A. Phenylketonuria
- B. Galactosemia
- C. Maple syrup urine disease
- D. Homocystinuria

Answer: B. Galactosemia

Explanation: In galactosemia, the accumulation of galactitol in the lens causes osmotic damage, resulting in early cataract formation. Other systemic effects include liver damage and intellectual disability.

Pearl: Lifelong dietary restriction of galactose is essential for preventing complications.

43. Which congenital anomaly can be treated with folic acid supplementation during pregnancy?

- A. Neural tube defects
- B. Cleft lip and palate
- C. Congenital diaphragmatic hernia
- D. Tetralogy of Fallot

Answer: A. Neural tube defects

Explanation: Adequate folic acid intake before conception and during early pregnancy significantly reduces the risk of neural tube defects such as spina bifida and anencephaly.

Pearl: Women of childbearing age should take 400–800 mcg of folic acid daily to prevent neural tube defects.

44. Which surgical intervention is performed to correct transposition of the great arteries (TGA)?

- A. Fontan procedure
- B. Arterial switch operation
- C. Blalock-Taussig shunt

- D. Norwood procedure

Answer: B. Arterial switch operation

Explanation: The arterial switch operation is the definitive surgical treatment for TGA, where the positions of the aorta and pulmonary artery are corrected to establish normal circulation.

Pearl: Early diagnosis and intervention, ideally within the first two weeks of life, are crucial for successful outcomes.

45. What is the preferred treatment for cleft palate in infants?

- A. Immediate surgical repair at birth
- B. Surgical repair between 9–18 months of age
- C. Use of a prosthetic obturator only
- D. Nutritional support without surgery

Answer: B. Surgical repair between 9–18 months of age

Explanation: Cleft palate repair is typically performed when the child is 9–18 months old to facilitate normal speech development and prevent feeding difficulties.

Pearl: Multidisciplinary care involving surgeons, speech therapists, and dentists is essential for optimal outcomes in cleft lip and palate management.

46. Which congenital anomaly can be treated with serial casting in infants?

- A. Congenital diaphragmatic hernia
- B. Gastroschisis
- C. Clubfoot (talipes equinovarus)
- D. Omphalocele

Answer: C. Clubfoot (talipes equinovarus)

Explanation: Serial casting, commonly using the Ponseti method, is the standard treatment for clubfoot. It involves weekly manipulation and casting to gradually correct the deformity.

Pearl: Early initiation of treatment within the first few weeks of life yields the best results.

47. Which vitamin supplementation can help prevent congenital anomalies like cleft lip and palate?

- A. Vitamin C
- B. Vitamin D
- C. Vitamin E
- D. Vitamin B complex, including folic acid

Answer: D. Vitamin B complex, including folic acid

Explanation: Adequate folic acid and vitamin B6 intake during pregnancy reduces the risk of cleft lip and palate, neural tube defects, and other congenital anomalies.

Pearl: Prenatal vitamins are recommended for all pregnant women to support healthy fetal development.

48. What is the definitive treatment for Hirschsprung disease?

- A. Serial enemas
- B. Dietary modification
- C. Surgical resection of the aganglionic segment
- D. Stoma placement without resection

Answer: C. Surgical resection of the aganglionic segment

Explanation: Hirschsprung disease is characterized by the absence of ganglion cells in the intestinal wall, leading to a functional obstruction. Surgical removal of the affected segment restores normal bowel function.

Pearl: Delayed diagnosis can result in severe complications such as enterocolitis.

49. What are inborn errors of metabolism (IEM)?

Answer: Inborn errors of metabolism are rare genetic disorders caused by defects in single genes that code for enzymes involved in metabolic processes. They result in the accumulation of toxic substances or the inability to synthesize essential compounds.

50. Name three examples of inborn errors of metabolism.
Answer. Three examples of inborn errors of metabolism are:

51. How are most inborn errors of metabolism diagnosed?
Answer: Most inborn errors of metabolism are diagnosed through newborn screening tests, which involve blood tests performed within hours of birth. Additional diagnostic methods include plasma amino acid tests, urine organic acid tests, and genetic testing

52: What are some common symptoms of inborn errors of metabolism?
Answer: Common symptoms of inborn errors of metabolism can include developmental delays, weight loss, growth challenges, seizures, poor appetite, lethargy, unusual odors in urine, sweat or breath, and abdominal pain

53: What are some treatment approaches for inborn errors of metabolism?
Answer: Treatment approaches for inborn errors of metabolism may include specialized diets designed by registered dietitians, enzyme replacement therapy, and management of acute metabolic crises. In some cases, vitamin or cofactor supplementation may be used

54. Which of the following is NOT a common feature of many inborn errors of metabolism?

a) Enzyme deficiency
b) Autosomal recessive inheritance
c) Accumulation of toxic metabolites
d) Autosomal dominant inheritance

Answer: d) Autosomal dominant inheritance

Explanation: Most inborn errors of metabolism are characterized by enzyme deficiencies, autosomal recessive inheritance, and the accumulation of toxic metabolites. Autosomal dominant inheritance is less common in these disorders.

55. In phenylketonuria (PKU), which enzyme is deficient?
a) Phenylalanine hydroxylase
b) Galactose-1-phosphate uridylyltransferase
c) Glucose-6-phosphatase
d) Medium-chain acyl-CoA dehydrogenase

Answer: a) Phenylalanine hydroxylase

Explanation: PKU is caused by a deficiency in phenylalanine hydroxylase, which normally converts phenylalanine to tyrosine. This deficiency leads to an accumulation of phenylalanine in the blood and tissues.

56. Which of the following is a key component in the management of many inborn errors of metabolism?
a) Antibiotic therapy
b) Dietary modification
c) Radiation therapy
d) Surgical intervention

Answer: b) Dietary modification

Explanation: Dietary modification is a crucial component in managing many inborn errors of metabolism. This often involves restricting the intake of certain nutrients that cannot be properly metabolized or supplementing with others that are deficient.

57.What is the primary goal of newborn screening for inborn errors of metabolism?
a) To cure the disorders
b) To prevent all symptoms
c) To identify and treat disorders before symptoms appear
d) To determine the prevalence of these disorders in the population

Answer: c) To identify and treat disorders before symptoms appear

Explanation: The main purpose of newborn screening is to identify infants with these disorders before they become symptomatic, allowing for early intervention and treatment to prevent or minimize complications.

58.Which of the following is a characteristic of organic acidemias?
a) Elevated blood glucose levels
b) Accumulation of organic acids in body fluids
c) Increased protein synthesis
d) Improved fatty acid oxidation

Answer: b) Accumulation of organic acids in body fluids

Explanation: Organic acidemias are a group of disorders characterized by the accumulation of organic acids in body fluids, particularly in the blood and urine. This accumulation is typically due to defects in enzymes involved in amino acid catabolism.

CONGENITAL CONDITIONS AND INBORN ERRORS OF METABOLISM

59.Which of the following is a primary goal of substrate reduction therapy (SRT) in inborn errors of metabolism?
a) Increasing enzyme production
b) Reducing the accumulation of toxic substrates
c) Replacing deficient enzymes
d) Enhancing metabolite production

Answer: b) Reducing the accumulation of toxic substrates

Explanation: Substrate reduction therapy (SRT) aims to decrease the production of toxic metabolites by inhibiting the enzyme responsible for their formation. This approach is particularly useful for intoxification-type inborn errors of metabolism where toxic metabolite accumulation leads to clinical symptoms

60.Enzyme replacement therapy (ERT) is most commonly used for which group of inborn errors of metabolism?
a) Urea cycle disorders
b) Lysosomal storage diseases
c) Fatty acid oxidation defects
d) Amino acid disorders

Answer: b) Lysosomal storage diseases

Explanation: Enzyme replacement therapy (ERT) is available for several lysosomal storage diseases, including Gaucher disease, Fabry disease, MPS I, MPS II (Hunter syndrome), MPS VI, and Pompe disease. ERT increases the concentration of the enzyme that the patient is lacking

61.Which of the following is NOT a common treatment strategy for inborn errors of metabolism?
a) Dietary modification

b) Enzyme replacement therapy
c) Radiation therapy
d) Pharmacological chaperone therapy

Answer: c) Radiation therapy

Explanation: Common treatment strategies for inborn errors of metabolism include dietary modification, enzyme replacement therapy, and pharmacological chaperone therapy. Radiation therapy is not typically used to treat these conditions

62.What is the primary advantage of small molecule therapies in treating inborn errors of metabolism with neurological involvement?
a) They are less expensive
b) They can potentially cross the blood-brain barrier
c) They have fewer side effects
d) They cure the underlying genetic defect

Answer: b) They can potentially cross the blood-brain barrier

Explanation: Small molecule therapies hold great promise for treating inborn errors of metabolism with neurological involvement because they can potentially cross the blood-brain barrier (BBB) to address CNS pathology, which is a limitation of some other treatment modalities

63.Which of the following is a key component of managing many inborn errors of metabolism diagnosed through newborn screening?
a) Immediate surgery
b) Early dietary intervention
c) Lifelong antibiotic therapy

d) Regular blood transfusions

Answer: b) Early dietary intervention

Explanation: For many inborn errors of metabolism diagnosed through newborn screening, early dietary intervention is crucial. Specialized diets created by registered dietitians can help prevent organ damage and other serious problems. These diets often need to be followed for life to manage the condition effectively

64.Which of the following is a common treatment approach for cleft lip and palate?
a) Medication only
b) Physical therapy
c) Surgical repair
d) Dietary modifications

Answer: c) Surgical repair

Explanation: Cleft lip and palate abnormalities are commonly treated by plastic surgeons who surgically repair the incomplete formation of the patient's upper lip or roof of the mouth

65.What is a potential benefit of fetal surgery for spina bifida?
a) Complete cure of the condition
b) Reduced risk of infection
c) Greater likelihood of walking without assistance
d) Elimination of all neurological deficits

Answer: c) Greater likelihood of walking without assistance

Explanation: The Management of Myelomeningocele

Study (MOMS) showed that fetal surgery for severe spina bifida greatly reduced health complications, including a greater likelihood of being able to walk without assistance

66. Which of the following is NOT a typical treatment modality for congenital heart defects in children?
a) Medications
b) Cardiac catheterization
c) Heart surgery
d) Radiation therapy

Answer: d) Radiation therapy

Explanation: Common treatments for congenital heart defects in children include medications, cardiac catheterization, and heart surgery. Radiation therapy is not typically used for treating congenital heart defects

67. When is pinna reconstruction typically performed for children with microtia?
a) Immediately after birth
b) At 2-3 years of age
c) At 6-7 years of age or later
d) Only in adulthood

Answer: c) At 6-7 years of age or later

Explanation: Pinna reconstruction requires harvesting sufficient autologous costal cartilage, which is not available until 6-7 years of age or so

68. Which of the following is a potential in-utero treatment for congenital diaphragmatic hernia?
a) Fetoscopic endotracheal occlusion
b) Amniocentesis
c) Cord blood transfusion

d) Maternal steroid therapy

Answer: a) Fetoscopic endotracheal occlusion

Explanation: Congenital diaphragmatic hernia can be significantly helped in utero through fetoscopic endotracheal occlusion, a surgery that improves lung function and significantly increases survival rates

69. Which of the following is considered the gold standard for invasive prenatal diagnosis in the first trimester?
a) Amniocentesis
b) Chorionic villus sampling (CVS)
c) Non-invasive prenatal testing (NIPT)
d) Maternal serum screening

Answer: b) Chorionic villus sampling (CVS)

Explanation: Chorionic villus sampling is the procedure of choice for invasive prenatal diagnosis in the first trimester, while mid-trimester amniocentesis is the most common form of invasive procedure for prenatal diagnosis

70. What percentage of central nervous system anomalies were found in the low-risk population at a specific institution in Turin?
a) 70%
b) 80%
c) 92%
d) 100%

Answer: c) 92%

Explanation: At the institution in Turin, 92% of 320 central nervous system anomalies prenatally detected over a 10-year period were found in the low-risk population

71. Which of the following is NOT a common prenatal screening method for congenital anomalies?
a) Ultrasound
b) Maternal serum biochemistry
c) X-ray
d) Non-invasive prenatal testing (NIPT)

Answer: c) X-ray

Explanation: Common prenatal screening methods include ultrasound, maternal serum biochemistry, and non-invasive prenatal testing. X-rays are not typically used for prenatal screening due to potential risks to the fetus

72. When is the first-trimester anatomical screening (FTAS) offered in the Netherlands?
a) Since 2007
b) Since 2015
c) Since September 2021
d) It is not offered

Answer: c) Since September 2021

Explanation: In the Netherlands, first-trimester anatomical screening (FTAS) has been offered since September 2021

73. Which of the following congenital anomalies is most commonly detected at birth rather than prenatally?
a) Neural tube defects
b) Cardiac malformations
c) Genital anomalies
d) Chromosomal abnormalities

Answer: c) Genital anomalies

Explanation: Genital anomalies, along with ear, face, neck, eye, and limb anomalies, are most commonly detected at birth. For instance, hypospadias, a common genital anomaly in male fetuses, is often difficult to detect prenatally and is frequently only identified at birth

74. Which of the following is considered a non-invasive prenatal test for genetic abnormalities?
a) Amniocentesis
b) Chorionic villus sampling
c) Cell-free DNA screening
d) Percutaneous umbilical blood sampling

Answer: c) Cell-free DNA screening

Explanation: Cell-free DNA screening is a non-invasive prenatal test that analyzes fragments of fetal DNA in maternal blood to screen for chromosomal abnormalities such as Down syndrome, trisomy 18, and trisomy 13

75. What is the primary advantage of the quadruple test in prenatal screening?
a) It can diagnose all genetic disorders
b) It predicts the chance of Down's syndrome
c) It is an invasive procedure
d) It is performed in the first trimester

Answer: b) It predicts the chance of Down's syndrome

Explanation: The quadruple test is mainly used to predict the chance of a baby having Down's syndrome by measuring the level of certain biochemical markers in the mother's blood sample

76. At which gestational age is amniocentesis typically performed?
a) 8-10 weeks
b) 11-13 weeks
c) 15 weeks or later
d) 30-32 weeks

Answer: c) 15 weeks or later

Explanation: Amniocentesis is usually done at 15 weeks of pregnancy or later. It involves removing a sample of amniotic fluid for analysis

77. Which of the following is NOT typically included in first trimester screening?
a) Maternal blood test
b) Ultrasound
c) Measurement of nuchal translucency
d) Fetal echocardiogram

Answer: d) Fetal echocardiogram

Explanation: First trimester screening typically includes a maternal blood test and an ultrasound that measures nuchal translucency. The fetal echocardiogram is usually performed during the second trimester ultrasound

78. Which of the following tests is considered a wide-net approach for diagnosing multiple inborn errors of metabolism?
a) Complete blood count
b) Liver function tests
c) Urine organic acid analysis
d) Electroencephalogram

Answer: c) Urine organic acid analysis

Explanation: Urine organic acid analysis is one of the laboratory tests that can be used to diagnose multiple inborn errors of metabolism, casting a wide net for potential disorders

79. What is the primary advantage of next-generation sequencing panels in diagnosing inborn errors of metabolism?
a) They are less expensive than biochemical tests
b) They can confirm diagnoses suggested by newborn screening
c) They eliminate the need for biochemical testing
d) They can only detect common mutations

Answer: b) They can confirm diagnoses suggested by newborn screening

Explanation: Extended next-generation sequencing panels can be used as a confirmatory test for suspected inborn errors of metabolism detected in newborn screening programs

80. Which of the following is NOT typically included in the minimal biochemical investigation for treatable inborn errors of metabolism?
a) Plasma amino acids
b) Urine organic acids
c) Acylcarnitine profile
d) Bone marrow biopsy

Answer: d) Bone marrow biopsy

Explanation: Minimal biochemical investigation to diagnose treatable inborn errors of metabolism typically includes tests like plasma amino acids, urine organic acids, and acylcarnitine profile, but not bone marrow biopsy

81. What is the purpose of the MARSALA technique in investigating inborn errors of metabolism?
a) To perform newborn screening
b) To conduct preimplantation genetic testing
c) To analyze urine metabolites
d) To measure enzyme activity

Answer: b) To conduct preimplantation genetic testing

Explanation: MARSALA (mutated allele revealed by sequencing with aneuploidy and linkage analyses) is used for preimplantation genetic testing for monogenic disorders (PGT-M) to prevent the transmission of inborn errors of metabolism

82. Which of the following statements about newborn screening for inborn errors of metabolism is correct?
a) It detects all possible inborn errors of metabolism
b) It may miss milder presentations of treatable disorders
c) It is only performed in high-risk pregnancies
d) It eliminates the need for further genetic testing

Answer: b) It may miss milder presentations of treatable disorders

Explanation: While newborn screening has advanced significantly, it may miss milder presentations of treatable inborn errors of metabolism, especially those with subtle biochemical phenotypes or milder mutations

83. Which of the following is a key advantage of tandem mass spectrometry (MS/MS) in newborn screening?
a) It can detect all known genetic mutations
b) It can screen for multiple disorders using a single blood

spot
c) It provides a definitive diagnosis without further testing
d) It eliminates false positive results completely

Answer: b) It can screen for multiple disorders using a single blood spot

Explanation: Tandem mass spectrometry (MS/MS) has revolutionized newborn screening by allowing for the simultaneous detection of multiple inborn errors of metabolism using a single blood spot, greatly expanding the number of disorders that can be screened.

84. What is the primary purpose of enzyme activity assays in diagnosing inborn errors of metabolism?
a) To identify genetic mutations
b) To measure the accumulation of metabolites
c) To directly assess the function of the affected enzyme
d) To determine the effectiveness of treatment

Answer: c) To directly assess the function of the affected enzyme

Explanation: Enzyme activity assays are used to directly measure the function of specific enzymes suspected to be deficient in certain inborn errors of metabolism, providing crucial diagnostic information.

85. Which of the following is NOT typically included in the initial evaluation of a neonate suspected of having an inborn error of metabolism?
a) Blood glucose
b) Serum electrolytes
c) Liver function tests
d) Whole genome sequencing

Answer: d) Whole genome sequencing

Explanation: Initial evaluation typically includes basic metabolic tests like blood glucose, serum electrolytes, and liver function tests. Whole genome sequencing, while potentially useful, is not part of the initial evaluation due to its cost and time requirements.

86. What is the main advantage of using dried blood spots in newborn screening?
a) They provide a complete genetic profile
b) They are easier to collect and transport than liquid blood samples
c) They eliminate the need for confirmatory testing
d) They can detect all possible metabolic disorders

Answer: b) They are easier to collect and transport than liquid blood samples

Explanation: Dried blood spots are widely used in newborn screening because they are easy to collect, require minimal blood volume, and can be easily transported and stored, making them ideal for large-scale screening programs.

87. Which of the following statements about whole exome sequencing (WES) in diagnosing inborn errors of metabolism is correct?
a) It always provides a definitive diagnosis
b) It can only detect known mutations
c) It can identify novel gene-disease associations
d) It is routinely used as a first-line diagnostic test

Answer: c) It can identify novel gene-disease associations

Explanation: Whole exome sequencing (WES) can be a powerful tool in diagnosing inborn errors of metabolism, particularly in complex cases. It has the potential to identify novel gene-disease associations, contributing to our understanding of these disorders.

88. Which of the following is a potential in-utero treatment for congenital diaphragmatic hernia?
a) Amniocentesis
b) Fetoscopic endotracheal occlusion
c) Cord blood transfusion
d) Maternal steroid therapy

Answer: b) Fetoscopic endotracheal occlusion

Explanation: Congenital diaphragmatic hernia can be significantly helped in utero through fetoscopic endotracheal occlusion, a surgery that improves lung function and significantly increases survival rates

89. What is a key advantage of cardiac catheterization in treating congenital heart defects in children?
a) It's less expensive than open-heart surgery
b) It can repair all types of heart defects
c) It allows for heart repair without open-heart surgery
d) It eliminates the need for follow-up care

Answer: c) It allows for heart repair without open-heart surgery

Explanation: Some types of congenital heart defects in children can be repaired using thin, flexible tubes called catheters. Such treatments let doctors fix the heart without open-heart surgery

**90. Which of the following medications is NOT typically

used to treat symptoms or complications of congenital heart defects?
a) ACE inhibitors
b) Beta blockers
c) Diuretics
d) Antibiotics

Answer: d) Antibiotics

Explanation: Medicines commonly used to treat congenital heart defects include blood pressure drugs (such as ACE inhibitors and beta blockers), diuretics, and anti-arrhythmic drugs. Antibiotics are not typically mentioned as a standard treatment for symptoms of congenital heart defects

91. Which of the following is a potential benefit of fetal surgery for spina bifida?
a) Complete cure of the condition
b) Reduced risk of infection
c) Greater likelihood of walking without assistance
d) Elimination of all neurological deficits

Answer: c) Greater likelihood of walking without assistance

Explanation: The Management of Myelomeningocele Study (MOMS) showed that fetal surgery for severe spina bifida greatly reduced health complications, including a greater likelihood of being able to walk without assistance

92. What is the estimated 20-year survival rate for individuals born with at least one congenital anomaly?
a) 75.5%
b) 80.5%

c) 85.5%
d) 90.5%

Answer: c) 85.5%

Explanation: According to a study, the 20-year survival rate for individuals born with at least one congenital anomaly was 85.5%

93. Which of the following congenital anomaly groups has the highest 20-year survival rate?
a) Cardiovascular system anomalies
b) Chromosomal anomalies
c) Urinary system anomalies
d) Nervous system anomalies

Answer: c) Urinary system anomalies

Explanation: The study reported a 20-year survival rate of 93.2% for urinary system anomalies, which is higher than the rates for cardiovascular system anomalies (89.5%), chromosomal anomalies (79.1%), and nervous system anomalies (66.2%)

94. What factor has been associated with improved survival rates for children with congenital anomalies over time?
a) Increased use of antibiotics
b) Higher rates of termination for fetal anomaly
c) Advancements in surgical techniques
d) Reduced environmental pollutants

Answer: b) Higher rates of termination for fetal anomaly

Explanation: The study found that the proportion of terminations for fetal anomaly increased throughout the study period and was an independent predictor of improved survival rates

95. Which of the following is NOT a common predictor of reduced survival for children with congenital anomalies?
a) Presence of additional structural anomalies
b) Low birth weight
c) Earlier year of birth
d) Higher maternal education level

Answer: d) Higher maternal education level

Explanation: The presence of additional structural anomalies, low birth weight, and earlier year of birth were the most commonly reported predictors of reduced survival for any congenital anomaly type

96. Up to what age has survival been shown to be decreased in patients with congenital heart defects?
a) 20 years
b) 30 years
c) 40 years
d) 50 years

Answer: c) 40 years

Explanation: A systematic review found that until the age of 40 years, survival is decreased in patients with congenital heart defects, although this is most pronounced among patients with complex heart defects

97. Which of the following is NOT typically included in the differential diagnosis for cyanotic congenital heart disease?
a) Pulmonary parenchymal disease

b) Sepsis
c) Hemoglobinopathy
d) Hypertension

Answer: d) Hypertension

Explanation: The differential diagnosis for cyanotic congenital heart disease typically includes pulmonary parenchymal disease, sepsis, and hemoglobinopathies (such as methemoglobinemia). Hypertension is not commonly associated with cyanosis in newborns

98. In the differential diagnosis of congenital heart defects, which of the following conditions is associated with increased pulmonary blood flow and cyanosis?
a) Ventricular septal defect
b) Tetralogy of Fallot
c) Transposition of great arteries
d) Coarctation of the aorta

Answer: c) Transposition of great arteries

Explanation: Transposition of great arteries is one of the cyanotic heart defects associated with increased pulmonary blood flow. It falls under the category of "admixture lesions" along with other conditions like total anomalous pulmonary venous return and truncus arteriosus

99. Which of the following tests is considered the definitive non-invasive test to determine the presence of congenital heart disease?
a) Electrocardiogram (ECG)
b) Chest X-ray
c) Two-dimensional echocardiography

d) Pulse oximetry screening

Answer: c) Two-dimensional echocardiography

Explanation: Two-dimensional echocardiography with Doppler is considered the definitive non-invasive test to determine the presence of congenital heart disease. It can determine the degree and direction of the shunt and the gradient of outflow tract obstruction

100. Which of the following is NOT one of the primary targets for critical congenital heart defect (CCHD) screening?
a) Hypoplastic left heart syndrome
b) Tetralogy of Fallot
c) Coarctation of the aorta
d) Total anomalous pulmonary venous return

Answer: c) Coarctation of the aorta

Explanation: While coarctation of the aorta is an important congenital heart defect, it is considered a secondary screening target for CCHD. The primary targets include hypoplastic left heart syndrome, tetralogy of Fallot, and total anomalous pulmonary venous return, among others

101. What is the purpose of the hyperoxia test in differentiating congenital heart disease from pulmonary disease?
a) To measure cardiac output
b) To assess pulmonary vascular resistance
c) To distinguish between cardiac and pulmonary causes of hypoxemia
d) To evaluate the severity of heart failure

CONGENITAL CONDITIONS AND INBORN ERRORS OF METABOLISM

Answer: c) To distinguish between cardiac and pulmonary causes of hypoxemia

Explanation: The hyperoxia test is used to distinguish congenital heart disease from pulmonary disease. In patients with congenital heart disease, PaO2 usually doesn't increase above 100 mmHg with 100% oxygen administration, while in pulmonary disease, PaO2 generally increases to ≥100 mmHg

102. Which of the following is NOT typically included in the differential diagnosis for a neonate presenting with acute metabolic encephalopathy?
a) Urea cycle defects
b) Organic acidemias
c) Nonketotic hyperglycinemia
d) Cystic fibrosis

Answer: d) Cystic fibrosis

Explanation: Urea cycle defects, organic acidemias, and nonketotic hyperglycinemia are common inborn errors of metabolism that can present with acute metabolic encephalopathy in neonates. Cystic fibrosis, while a genetic disorder, does not typically cause acute metabolic encephalopathy

103. In differentiating between metabolic disorders and sepsis in a neonate, which of the following is more suggestive of an inborn error of metabolism?
a) Presence of fever
b) Neutropenia
c) Hyperammonemia
d) Positive blood culture

Answer: c) Hyperammonemia

Explanation: While sepsis may be the initial consideration in a neonate with acute symptoms, hyperammonemia is more suggestive of an inborn error of metabolism, particularly urea cycle defects or certain organic acidemias

104. Which of the following conditions should be considered in the differential diagnosis of an infant presenting with hypoglycemia?
a) Glycogen storage disorders
b) Fatty acid oxidation defects
c) Defects in gluconeogenesis
d) All of the above

Answer: d) All of the above

Explanation: Hypoglycemia may be the predominant finding in several inborn errors of metabolism, including glycogen storage disorders, defects in gluconeogenesis, and fatty acid oxidation defects

105. Which of the following is NOT typically associated with metabolic acidosis in inborn errors of metabolism?
a) Organic acidemias
b) Mitochondrial disorders
c) Urea cycle defects
d) Fatty acid oxidation defects

Answer: c) Urea cycle defects

Explanation: Metabolic acidosis is commonly observed in organic acidemias, mitochondrial disorders, and fatty acid oxidation defects. Urea cycle defects typically present with hyperammonemia without significant metabolic acidosis

CONGENITAL CONDITIONS AND INBORN ERRORS OF METABOLISM

106. **Which congenital anomaly commonly causes neonatal respiratory distress and requires emergency intervention?**
- A. Congenital diaphragmatic hernia
- B. Duodenal atresia
- C. Tracheoesophageal fistula
- D. Omphalocele

Answer: A. Congenital diaphragmatic hernia

Explanation: Congenital diaphragmatic hernia (CDH) involves herniation of abdominal contents into the thoracic cavity, impairing lung development and causing respiratory distress. Emergency stabilization and surgical repair are essential.

Pearl: Prenatal diagnosis and delivery at a tertiary care center improve outcomes in CDH.

107. **What is the immediate management priority for a neonate born with gastroschisis?**
- A. Surgical repair within 24 hours
- B. Protecting the exposed bowel with sterile covering and temperature regulation
- C. Initiating total parenteral nutrition
- D. Intubation and mechanical ventilation

Answer: B. Protecting the exposed bowel with sterile covering and temperature regulation

Explanation: In gastroschisis, the bowel is exposed and prone to injury and infection. Sterile covering, thermoregulation, and fluid resuscitation are crucial before definitive surgical repair.

Pearl: Prompt transfer to a neonatal surgical unit improves survival in gastroschisis.

108. **Which emergency intervention is critical in the management of a neonate with tracheoesophageal fistula (TEF)?**
- A. Immediate surgical repair

- B. Prevention of aspiration by positioning and suctioning
- C. Insertion of a nasogastric tube
- D. Administration of broad-spectrum antibiotics

Answer: B. Prevention of aspiration by positioning and suctioning

Explanation: TEF often leads to aspiration and respiratory distress. Immediate prevention of aspiration with positioning and suctioning is critical, followed by surgical repair.

Pearl: Early recognition of TEF prevents complications like pneumonia and sepsis.

109. Which congenital cardiac anomaly requires prostaglandin E1 infusion as an emergency treatment?

- A. Hypoplastic left heart syndrome
- B. Tetralogy of Fallot
- C. Ventricular septal defect
- D. Patent ductus arteriosus

Answer: A. Hypoplastic left heart syndrome

Explanation: Prostaglandin E1 maintains ductal patency, ensuring systemic circulation in neonates with hypoplastic left heart syndrome until surgical intervention can be performed.

Pearl: Early initiation of prostaglandin E1 improves outcomes in duct-dependent cardiac anomalies.

110. What is the hallmark clinical presentation of an infant with intestinal malrotation and volvulus?

- A. Failure to pass meconium
- B. Bilious vomiting and abdominal distension
- C. Non-bilious vomiting and jaundice
- D. Cyanosis and apnea

Answer: B. Bilious vomiting and abdominal distension

CONGENITAL CONDITIONS AND INBORN ERRORS OF METABOLISM

Explanation: Intestinal malrotation with volvulus presents with bilious vomiting, abdominal pain, and distension, requiring urgent surgical intervention to prevent bowel necrosis.

Pearl: Bilious vomiting in neonates is a surgical emergency until proven otherwise.

111. What is the first-line imaging study for suspected congenital pyloric stenosis?
- A. Abdominal X-ray
- B. Ultrasound
- C. Upper GI contrast study
- D. CT scan

Answer: B. Ultrasound

Explanation: Ultrasound is the diagnostic modality of choice for pyloric stenosis, showing hypertrophy of the pyloric muscle.

Pearl: Prompt recognition and correction of dehydration and electrolyte imbalances precede surgical management.

112. Which surgical emergency is commonly associated with omphalocele?
- A. Cardiac defects
- B. Neural tube defects
- C. Renal agenesis
- D. Cleft palate

Answer: A. Cardiac defects

Explanation: Omphalocele often coexists with other anomalies, particularly cardiac defects, necessitating a thorough preoperative evaluation.

Pearl: Multidisciplinary care improves outcomes in neonates with omphalocele.

113. What is the most common cause of cyanosis in a newborn requiring emergency intervention?

- A. Atrial septal defect
- B. Tetralogy of Fallot
- C. Transposition of the great arteries
- D. Coarctation of the aorta

Answer: C. Transposition of the great arteries

Explanation: Transposition of the great arteries results in severe cyanosis due to parallel circulation. Emergency prostaglandin E1 infusion and balloon atrial septostomy are lifesaving.

Pearl: Early recognition and intervention are critical in cyanotic congenital heart disease.

114. **Which chromosomal abnormality is associated with a single palmar crease and congenital heart defects?**
     - A. Trisomy 21
     - B. Trisomy 18
     - C. Trisomy 13
     - D. Turner syndrome

Answer: A. Trisomy 21

Explanation: Trisomy 21 (Down syndrome) is associated with distinctive physical features, including a single palmar crease, intellectual disability, and congenital heart defects like atrioventricular septal defect (AVSD).

Pearl: Prenatal screening with nuchal translucency and non-invasive prenatal testing (NIPT) can identify the risk of trisomy 21.

115. **What is the characteristic hand position seen in Trisomy 18 (Edward syndrome)?**
     - A. Clenched fists with overlapping fingers
     - B. Widened first and second toes
     - C. Clinodactyly of the fifth finger
     - D. Polydactyly

Answer: A. Clenched fists with overlapping fingers

CONGENITAL CONDITIONS AND INBORN ERRORS OF METABOLISM

Explanation: Trisomy 18 is associated with clenched fists, overlapping fingers, and other anomalies such as rocker-bottom feet and cardiac defects.

Pearl: Trisomy 18 has a poor prognosis with high neonatal mortality.

116. Which trisomy is associated with holoprosencephaly, microphthalmia, and cleft lip/palate?

- A. Trisomy 13
- B. Trisomy 21
- C. Trisomy 18
- D. Turner syndrome

Answer: A. Trisomy 13

Explanation: Trisomy 13 (Patau syndrome) often presents with midline facial defects, severe intellectual disability, and holoprosencephaly due to abnormal forebrain development.

Pearl: Early diagnosis allows for informed decision-making and supportive care.

117. What is the most common cardiac defect in Turner syndrome?

- A. Coarctation of the aorta
- B. Atrial septal defect
- C. Tetralogy of Fallot
- D. Ventricular septal defect

Answer: A. Coarctation of the aorta

Explanation: Turner syndrome (45, X) is frequently associated with coarctation of the aorta, as well as other anomalies like bicuspid aortic valve and short stature.

Pearl: Lymphedema at birth may suggest Turner syndrome.

118. Which chromosomal abnormality is associated with

gynecomastia, small testes, and tall stature in males?

- A. Klinefelter syndrome
- B. Turner syndrome
- C. Trisomy 21
- D. XYY syndrome

Answer: A. Klinefelter syndrome

Explanation: Klinefelter syndrome (47, XXY) is characterized by hypogonadism, infertility, and gynecomastia. Testosterone replacement therapy is often needed.

Pearl: Early diagnosis and hormonal therapy improve quality of life.

119.**What prenatal diagnostic technique is most definitive for detecting chromosomal abnormalities?**

- A. Maternal serum screening
- B. Amniocentesis
- C. Ultrasound
- D. Fetal MRI

Answer: B. Amniocentesis

Explanation: Amniocentesis allows for karyotyping or chromosomal microarray analysis to detect chromosomal abnormalities definitively.

Pearl: Chorionic villus sampling (CVS) is another invasive option but is done earlier in pregnancy.

120.**What genetic condition is associated with large ears, macroorchidism, and intellectual disability?**

- A. Fragile X syndrome
- B. Trisomy 21
- C. Turner syndrome
- D. Klinefelter syndrome

Answer: A. Fragile X syndrome

Explanation: Fragile X syndrome, caused by a CGG repeat expansion in the FMR1 gene, is the most common inherited cause of intellectual disability in males.

Pearl: Testing for FMR1 mutation is essential in cases of unexplained developmental delay.

121. What is the characteristic finding on ultrasound for fetuses with trisomy 21?

- A. Omphalocele
- B. Enlarged bladder
- C. Increased nuchal translucency
- D. Rocker-bottom feet

Answer: C. Increased nuchal translucency

Explanation: Increased nuchal translucency (NT) on first-trimester ultrasound is a key marker for trisomy 21 and other chromosomal abnormalities.

Pearl: NT measurements are part of first-trimester screening alongside biochemical markers.

122. What is the recurrence risk of trisomy 21 in subsequent pregnancies after one affected child?

- A. 1-2%
- B. 1% above maternal age-related risk
- C. 10%
- D. 25%

Answer: B. 1% above maternal age-related risk

Explanation: The recurrence risk of trisomy 21 is slightly higher than the age-related risk, depending on whether it resulted from nondisjunction or translocation.

Pearl: Genetic counseling is essential for families with a history of chromosomal abnormalities.

123. What is the major cause of death in infants with Trisomy 18?

- A. Sepsis
- B. Congenital heart defects
- C. Renal failure
- D. Neurological complications

Answer: B. Congenital heart defects

Explanation: Congenital heart defects, particularly ventricular septal defects and atrial septal defects, are the leading cause of mortality in Trisomy 18.

Pearl: Supportive care and palliative interventions are often required in Trisomy 18.

124. Which chromosomal abnormality is associated with a webbed neck and a wide carrying angle?
- A. Turner syndrome
- B. Trisomy 13
- C. Klinefelter syndrome
- D. Fragile X syndrome

Answer: A. Turner syndrome

Explanation: Turner syndrome presents with characteristic physical features, including a webbed neck, lymphedema, and cubitus valgus.

Pearl: Early estrogen therapy can aid in achieving secondary sexual development.

125. What is the most common karyotype in Down syndrome?
- A. Non-disjunction of chromosome 21
- B. Robertsonian translocation
- C. Mosaicism
- D. Trisomy 18

Answer: A. Non-disjunction of chromosome 21

Explanation: Non-disjunction during meiosis is the most common cause of Down syndrome, accounting for approximately

95% of cases.

Pearl: Advanced maternal age is a significant risk factor for non-disjunction.

126. Which chromosomal abnormality is associated with cat-like crying in infants?
- A. Cri du chat syndrome
- B. Trisomy 21
- C. Trisomy 18
- D. Angelman syndrome

Answer: A. Cri du chat syndrome

Explanation: Cri du chat syndrome results from a deletion on chromosome 5p, characterized by a high-pitched cry, microcephaly, and developmental delay.

Pearl: Chromosomal microarray testing is diagnostic for microdeletions.

127. What laboratory test is recommended for prenatal screening of trisomy 21?
- A. Karyotyping
- B. Non-invasive prenatal testing (NIPT)
- C. FISH analysis
- D. Chromosomal microarray

Answer: B. Non-invasive prenatal testing (NIPT)

Explanation: NIPT analyzes cell-free fetal DNA and is highly sensitive and specific for detecting trisomies.

Pearl: NIPT can be performed as early as 10 weeks of gestation.

128. What is the characteristic facial feature of a child with Trisomy 21?
- A. High forehead
- B. Macroglossia
- C. Epicanthic folds

- D. Small ears

Answer: C. Epicanthic folds

Explanation: Trisomy 21 is associated with epicanthic folds, upslanting palpebral fissures, and a flat nasal bridge.

Pearl: Multidisciplinary care is vital for managing comorbidities in Down syndrome.

129. What is the most common clinical presentation of talipes equinovarus (clubfoot)?

- A. Dorsiflexion of the ankle with eversion of the foot
- B. Plantar flexion of the ankle with inversion of the foot
- C. Neutral ankle position with external rotation of the foot
- D. Plantar flexion of the ankle with eversion of the foot

Answer: B. Plantar flexion of the ankle with inversion of the foot

Explanation: Talipes equinovarus is characterized by plantar flexion (equinus), inversion (varus), and adduction of the forefoot.

Pearl: Early diagnosis and treatment with serial casting (e.g., Ponseti method) are critical to achieving optimal outcomes.

130. Which of the following conditions is most commonly associated with congenital talipes equinovarus?

- A. Spina bifida
- B. Trisomy 21
- C. Congenital diaphragmatic hernia
- D. Turner syndrome

Answer: A. Spina bifida

Explanation: Talipes equinovarus is frequently associated with neural tube defects, such as spina bifida, due to abnormal neuromuscular development.

Pearl: Neurological evaluation is essential in infants with clubfoot to rule out underlying spinal or neuromuscular conditions.

131. Which of the following is a hallmark clinical feature of mitochondrial disorders?

- A. Isolated hyperglycemia
- B. Recurrent otitis media
- C. Multisystem involvement with lactic acidosis
- D. Hypothyroidism

Answer: C. Multisystem involvement with lactic acidosis

Explanation: Mitochondrial disorders typically present with multisystem involvement, reflecting defects in energy production. Lactic acidosis is a hallmark feature due to impaired oxidative phosphorylation. Commonly affected systems include the nervous system, muscles, and eyes.

Pearl: A high index of suspicion is required for early diagnosis, particularly in patients with unexplained lactic acidosis.

132. What is the inheritance pattern most commonly associated with mitochondrial disorders?

- A. Autosomal recessive
- B. Autosomal dominant
- C. X-linked
- D. Maternal inheritance

Answer: D. Maternal inheritance

Explanation: Mitochondrial DNA is exclusively inherited from the mother, and mutations in mitochondrial DNA lead to a maternal inheritance pattern. However, nuclear DNA mutations affecting mitochondria may follow

Mendelian inheritance.

Pearl: Detailed family history is crucial for identifying maternal transmission in suspected cases.

133. Which diagnostic test is most definitive for confirming a mitochondrial disorder?

- A. Serum lactate and pyruvate ratio
- B. MRI of the brain
- C. Muscle biopsy with electron transport chain studies
- D. Genetic testing

Answer: D. Genetic testing

Explanation: While muscle biopsy and metabolic studies are helpful, genetic testing of mitochondrial and nuclear DNA provides a definitive diagnosis, identifying specific mutations.

Pearl: Whole-exome sequencing can be valuable when initial targeted genetic tests are inconclusive.

134. Which syndrome is a classic example of a mitochondrial disorder?

- A. Marfan syndrome
- B. Rett syndrome
- C. MELAS syndrome
- D. Guillain-Barré syndrome

Answer: C. MELAS syndrome

Explanation: MELAS (Mitochondrial Encephalopathy, Lactic Acidosis, and Stroke-like episodes) is a well-known mitochondrial disorder characterized by neurological and systemic manifestations, including stroke-like episodes and progressive cognitive decline.

Pearl: Early recognition and management can help mitigate stroke-like episodes and associated complications.

135. What is the gold standard for diagnosing Gaucher disease?

- A. Bone marrow biopsy
- B. Genetic testing for GBA mutations
- C. Measurement of glucocerebrosidase activity
- D. Plasma chitotriosidase levels

Answer: C. Measurement of glucocerebrosidase activity

Explanation: The definitive diagnosis of Gaucher disease is made by measuring glucocerebrosidase enzyme activity in leukocytes or cultured fibroblasts. Genetic testing and plasma biomarkers like chitotriosidase are supportive but not definitive.

Pearl: Early diagnosis through enzyme activity assays allows timely intervention with ERT or substrate reduction therapy.

136.. Which of the following is a common skeletal manifestation of Gaucher disease?

- A. Osteoporosis
- B. Erlenmeyer flask deformity of the femur
- C. Lytic bone lesions
- D. All of the above

Answer: D. All of the above

Explanation: Skeletal complications in Gaucher disease include osteoporosis, characteristic Erlenmeyer flask deformities (due to abnormal bone modeling), and lytic lesions leading to bone pain and fractures.

Pearl: Regular monitoring of bone health and density is crucial in managing Gaucher disease.

137.. Which type of Gaucher disease is most severe and associated with early neurological involvement?

- A. Type 1 (non-neuropathic)
- B. Type 2 (acute neuropathic)
- C. Type 3 (chronic neuropathic)
- D. Perinatal lethal Gaucher disease

Answer: B. Type 2 (acute neuropathic)

Explanation: Type 2 Gaucher disease is the most severe form, characterized by early onset, progressive neurological decline, and a poor prognosis. Unlike Type 1, it involves the central nervous system.

Pearl: Type 2 Gaucher disease lacks effective treatment options, highlighting the need for genetic counseling in affected families.

138. Which of the following is a treatment approach for mitochondrial disorders?
    - A. Gene therapy
    - B. High-dose steroids
    - C. Supportive care and coenzyme Q10 supplementation
    - D. Antiviral therapy

Answer: C. Supportive care and coenzyme Q10 supplementation

Explanation: Treatment for mitochondrial disorders is largely supportive, focusing on optimizing energy metabolism. Coenzyme Q10, a mitochondrial cofactor, may provide symptomatic relief in some cases.

Pearl: Avoiding mitochondrial toxins like valproic acid and ensuring adequate nutrition are essential components of management.

139. What is the primary treatment for congenital talipes equinovarus in the neonatal period?
    - A. Surgical correction at birth
    - B. Physiotherapy alone
    - C. Serial casting with the Ponseti method
    - D. Use of orthotic braces only

Answer: C. Serial casting with the Ponseti method

Explanation: The Ponseti method is the gold standard for

CONGENITAL CONDITIONS AND INBORN ERRORS OF METABOLISM

treating congenital talipes equinovarus. It involves gentle manipulation and weekly casting to gradually correct the deformity.

Pearl: Surgical intervention is reserved for cases resistant to conservative management.

140. Which imaging modality is most useful in diagnosing talipes equinovarus prenatally?

- A. MRI
- B. Ultrasound
- C. CT scan
- D. X-ray

Answer: B. Ultrasound

Explanation: Prenatal ultrasound can detect talipes equinovarus by visualizing the abnormal position of the fetal foot.

Pearl: Prenatal detection allows for early parental counseling and planning postnatal treatment strategies.

141. What is the most common complication associated with untreated congenital talipes equinovarus?

- A. Frequent fractures of the lower limb
- B. Chronic pain and difficulty walking
- C. Limb length discrepancy
- D. Hip dysplasia

Answer: B. Chronic pain and difficulty walking

Explanation: Untreated clubfoot can lead to significant functional impairment, including difficulty walking and chronic pain due to joint and muscle imbalances.

Pearl: Early intervention with non-surgical methods is critical to prevent long-term complications.

142. What is the primary biochemical defect in Gaucher disease?

- A. Deficiency of alpha-galactosidase A
- B. Deficiency of glucocerebrosidase

- C. Deficiency of sphingomyelinase
- D. Deficiency of iduronidase

Answer: B. Deficiency of glucocerebrosidase

Explanation: Gaucher disease results from a deficiency of the lysosomal enzyme glucocerebrosidase, leading to the accumulation of glucocerebroside in macrophages. This results in the formation of Gaucher cells, which are characteristic lipid-laden macrophages.

Pearl: Enzyme replacement therapy (ERT) is the mainstay of treatment for certain types of Gaucher disease.

143. Which clinical feature is least likely to be seen in Gaucher disease?

- A. Hepatosplenomegaly
- B. Pancytopenia
- C. Bone crises
- D. Cherry-red spot on the macula

Answer: D. Cherry-red spot on the macula

Explanation: While hepatosplenomegaly, pancytopenia, and bone crises are common in Gaucher disease, a cherry-red spot on the macula is more characteristic of Tay-Sachs disease or Niemann-Pick disease.

Pearl: Always correlate clinical findings with specific lysosomal storage diseases to avoid misdiagnosis.

144. Which of the following best describes the anatomical defect in hypospadias?

- A. Ventral displacement of the urethral meatus
- B. Dorsal displacement of the urethral meatus
- C. Urethral stricture in the posterior urethra
- D. Absence of the urethral meatus

Answer: A. Ventral displacement of the urethral meatus

Explanation:

Hypospadias is characterized by the urethral opening being located on the ventral (underside) aspect of the penis, often accompanied by a ventral curvature (chordee) and incomplete foreskin formation.

Pearl: Early surgical repair, usually between 6 to 12 months of age, improves both cosmetic and functional outcomes.

145.. Which associated condition is most frequently seen in infants with hypospadias?
- A. Vesicoureteral reflux
- B. Cryptorchidism
- C. Posterior urethral valves
- D. Horseshoe kidney

Answer: B. Cryptorchidism

Explanation:
Cryptorchidism (undescended testes) is commonly associated with hypospadias, especially in severe cases. The presence of both conditions may warrant evaluation for disorders of sexual development.

Pearl: In cases of hypospadias with cryptorchidism, a karyotype and hormonal evaluation may be necessary to rule out intersex conditions.

146.. What is the primary goal of surgical correction in hypospadias?
- A. Improve cosmetic appearance of the penis
- B. Prevent recurrent urinary tract infections
- C. Achieve a straight penis with a functionally normal urethra
- D. Address associated cryptorchidism

Answer: C. Achieve a straight penis with a functionally normal urethra

Explanation:
The primary goals of surgical correction are to create a straight

penis (by correcting chordee), construct a urethra that allows normal voiding and ejaculation, and improve the cosmetic appearance of the penis.

Pearl: The timing of surgery is typically before 18 months of age to minimize psychological impact and maximize functional outcomes.

147. Which congenital heart defect is characterized by a continuous "machine-like" murmur on auscultation?

- A. Atrial septal defect (ASD)
- B. Ventricular septal defect (VSD)
- C. Patent ductus arteriosus (PDA)
- D. Tetralogy of Fallot

Answer: C. Patent ductus arteriosus (PDA)

Explanation:
A patent ductus arteriosus leads to a continuous "machine-like" murmur, heard best at the left infraclavicular area. It results from persistent blood flow between the aorta and pulmonary artery.

Pearl: Indomethacin or ibuprofen is used to close a PDA in preterm infants, while surgical or catheter-based closure may be needed in term infants and older children.

148. What is the most common congenital heart defect in Down syndrome?

- A. Atrioventricular septal defect (AVSD)
- B. Tetralogy of Fallot
- C. Coarctation of the aorta
- D. Pulmonary stenosis

Answer: A. Atrioventricular septal defect (AVSD)

Explanation:
AVSD is the most common congenital heart defect in individuals with Down syndrome, caused by incomplete fusion of the endocardial cushions, resulting in a combination of ASD and VSD.

Pearl: Early surgical repair is essential to prevent pulmonary hypertension and improve long-term outcomes.

149. Which of the following is NOT a component of Tetralogy of Fallot?

- A. Right ventricular hypertrophy
- B. Pulmonary stenosis
- C. Left ventricular outflow tract obstruction
- D. Ventricular septal defect

Answer: C. Left ventricular outflow tract obstruction

Explanation:
Tetralogy of Fallot includes four components: right ventricular hypertrophy, pulmonary stenosis, a ventricular septal defect, and overriding aorta. Left ventricular outflow tract obstruction is not part of this condition.

Pearl: Cyanotic spells ("Tet spells") in Tetralogy of Fallot can be managed acutely by placing the child in a knee-chest position to increase systemic vascular resistance.

150. What is the primary defect in Zellweger syndrome?

- A. Deficiency of lysosomal enzymes
- B. Impaired mitochondrial DNA repair
- C. Failure to form functional peroxisomes
- D. Decreased glycolysis in the cytoplasm

Answer: C. Failure to form functional peroxisomes

Explanation:
Zellweger syndrome is a peroxisomal biogenesis disorder caused by mutations in PEX genes, leading to the absence of functional peroxisomes. This results in the accumulation of very-long-chain fatty acids (VLCFAs) and other toxic metabolites.

Pearl: Zellweger syndrome typically presents with severe hypotonia, craniofacial abnormalities, seizures, and early death.

151. Which of the following is a characteristic biochemical finding in peroxisomal disorders like Zellweger syndrome?

- A. Elevated glucose levels

- B. Elevated very-long-chain fatty acids (VLCFAs)
- C. Decreased serum lactate levels
- D. Increased pyruvate dehydrogenase activity

Answer: B. Elevated very-long-chain fatty acids (VLCFAs)

Explanation:

Peroxisomes are essential for the breakdown of VLCFAs. In disorders like Zellweger syndrome, defective peroxisomal function leads to the accumulation of VLCFAs, a hallmark diagnostic finding.

Pearl: VLCFA levels can be measured in plasma for diagnosis, and genetic testing confirms the specific peroxisomal biogenesis defect.

ABOUT THE AUTHOR

Dr Essam Abdelhakim

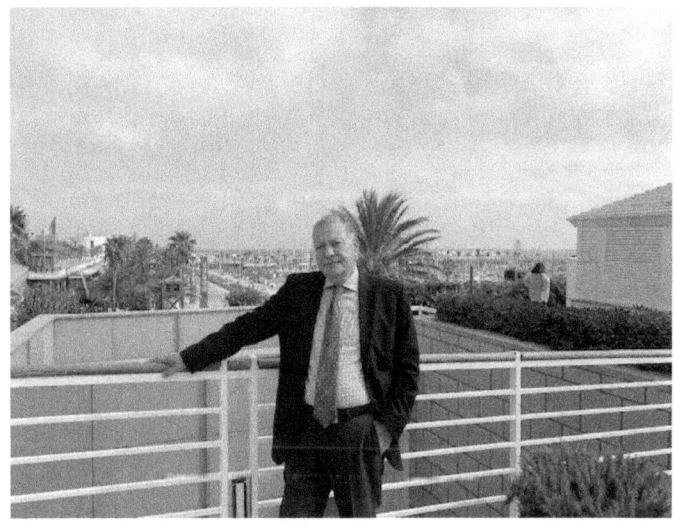

Senior consultant and Expert in Medical Education

www.ingramcontent.com/pod-product-compliance
Lightning Source LLC
Chambersburg PA
CBHW070409230526
45471CB00006B/2724